PILGRIMAGE

*A guide for the journey
of pain and healing*

MICHAEL STAHL

For the millions suffering from chronic pain, the search for effective treatment options seems like a minefield. There are so many different opinions, so many different types of providers, so many "quick-fix" promises...and yet it all still ends up confusing, inaccessible, or out-of-reach for all involved. Frustrated patients and providers desperately need a framework to understand and navigate this complex experience of healing from both sides. I am a board-certified anesthesiologist and pain physician, having trained and worked at some of the most reputable institutions in the country; I have gotten additional certification in acupuncture and yoga; I have lectured to providers and listened to patients both here and abroad; I have started holistic retreats and non-profit organizations to better advocate for integrated pain management. Yet "Pilgrimage" is the first book I've read that truly captures both the essence AND practicality of what it really takes for true healing. Michael Stahl combines neuroscience and common sense, anecdote and reference, theory and practice, for provider and patient. He takes his personal and professional background with chronic pain and translates it—simply and elegantly—into a universal tool every single person can use. Importantly, it doesn't promote any one type of treatment paradigm or focus on any one type of pain; his message is applicable to all of us, no matter our place in our own pilgrimage. A must read.

—Tracy Jackson, MD
Associate Professor of Anesthesiology and Pain Medicine, Vanderbilt University
CEO, Relief Retreats; Founder, camPAIN.org

Being a witness to someone's journey and being trusted to be present with them on that journey is a tremendous privilege and honor. Michael has given me that privilege. Within these pages, he has captured what I have seen change lives over and over again. His ability to assimilate multiple layers of information and perspective into a clear, understandable picture is part of his genius. As you walk this pilgrimage, know you are following a path that Michael not only understands but has also walked himself. A gift he offers is for you to traverse your own pilgrimage into your own life and body, finding a way amongst the valleys and the vistas.

– Mindy Oldham, RN, LMT
Director of Clinical Education, Instructor of Integrative Therapy
Cumberland Institute of Holistic Therapies

ISBN-13: 978-1540484659
ISBN-10: 1540484653

First Edition

Design by Tim Delger

To Mindy Oldham and Mary Beth Crawford—for having the courage to walk your own journeys and share your experience...showing so many people, including me, what is possible.

—MGS

PILGRIMAGE...

"...a transformative journey to a sacred center full of hardships, darkness, and peril. In the tradition of pilgrimage, those hardships are seen not as accidental, but as integral to the journey itself. Treacherous terrain, bad weather, taking a fall, getting lost—challenges of that sort, largely beyond our control, can strip the ego of the illusion that it is in charge and make space for true self to emerge. If that happens, the pilgrim has a better chance to find the sacred center he or she seeks. Disabused of our illusions by much travel and travail, we awaken one day to find that the sacred center is here and now—in every moment of the journey, everywhere in the world around us, and deep within our own hearts."

Parker Palmer, *Let Your Life Speak*, pg. 18. Josey-Bass, 2000.

Contents

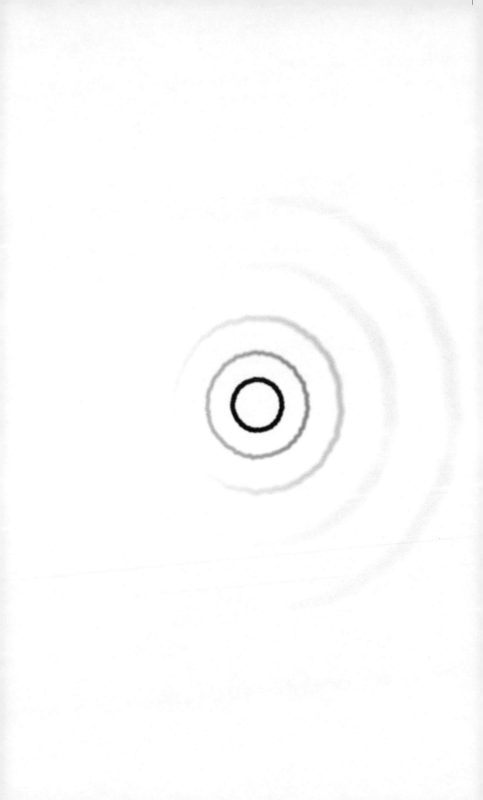

"I FEEL BROKEN."

I've heard countless clients say it when they first come to my office. Desperate to get relief from pain. Frustrated at all the time and money they feel they've wasted getting scans and talking to experts—without change. Feeling lost and helpless since they cannot find a path to relief.

I understand. I have felt broken, too—like my body was failing me. Like I could not regain the ability to move through my daily life as I tried to recover from a broken back and two hip surgeries.

I continued to feel broken and struggle until I began to understand how we, as humans, experience pain and what we need to heal. As I gained a deeper understanding of the mechanisms underlying pain and the healing process, I began to see that I was not broken. Rather, the pain and tension I experienced were actually information designed to protect me from further harm. These symptoms I had fought so hard to suppress or avoid were actually signs that my body was resilient and functioning exactly as it was designed.

I just needed to understand how it was protecting me so that I could work with my body rather than against it.

As I dug deeper into fields such as neuroscience, physical therapy, and other healing arts from the East and West, I began to notice a common framework for pain and healing. As my understanding solidified, I began to follow this framework—noticing that my healing accelerated and deepened if I could follow it rather than fight against it.

I then took this framework and combined the theory of pain and healing with practical techniques I could incorporate into my daily life—both for my own recovery and the recovery of my clients.

As I began to apply it to my work with clients, I noticed they experienced similar results to mine. I noticed that my clients' healing seemed to deepen when our work honored the healing process laid out in this workbook. As they followed the framework, they deepened their understanding of themselves, their pain, and how to enhance their own healing and sense of wellness.

They shifted:

- **From feeling broken to resilient:** Understanding pain as a natural, adaptive human response to injury, trauma, and/or instability reflects a natural survival response to a stimulus that we perceive as unsafe. Our bodies are not broken; they are incredibly resilient and help us survive.

- **From fixing their body to facilitating healing:** If nothing is broken, nothing needs to be fixed. Healing involves becoming more attuned with how we perceive our environment as unsafe so that we can understand how our bodies are trying to protect us and what we need to heal. In order to facilitate, we need to listen and respond to what our bodies have to say.

- **From feeling helpless to empowered:** With awareness comes the ability to make an informed decision about how to engage with that pain and vulnerability. Regardless of the course of action, when you can make that informed decision, you can again participate actively in your own healing and wellness.

- **From avoiding pain and tension to engaging them:** Rather than viewing pain, tension, and other challenges as something to suppress or eliminate, we understand that healing comes from safely engaging with that vulnerability to move through it and process it.

I created this workbook to share the information I provide my clients with a broader audience. As with my clients, the information in this workbook is designed to support your healing process. To help explain and reframe how our bodies and minds experience pain and healing. To help you use this understanding to inform how you approach your own healing so that you may be able to engage with the pain and vulnerability in a safe, productive manner.

I call this a pilgrimage because it is not easy. As Parker Palmer said, a pilgrimage is:

> ...a transformative journey to a sacred center full of hardships, darkness, and peril. In the tradition of pilgrimage, those hardships are seen not as accidental, but as integral to the journey itself. Treacherous terrain, bad weather, taking a fall, getting lost—challenges of that sort, largely beyond our control, can strip the ego of the illusion that it is in charge and make space for true self to emerge. If that happens, the pilgrim has a better chance to find the sacred center he or she seeks. Disabused of our illusions by much travel and travail, we awaken one day to find that the sacred center is here and now—in every moment of the journey, everywhere in the world around us, and deep within our own hearts.

> —Parker Palmer, *Let Your Life Speak*, pg. 18. Josey-Bass, 2000.

As Palmer notes, these challenges you experience—the pain, the tension, the unknown—are the keys to your healing and growth. It's just knowing how to listen and how to engage them safely, which can be particularly challenging when pain or tension has you feeling broken, desperate, and lost.

It is my deep honor to share this information with you. I hope that you can use this workbook to support yourself as you walk through your own healing pilgrimage. I have tried to distill my education, training, and experience into a clear framework that can help serve as a resource, a sort of compass, to help you orient yourself during this process that can be challenging and fraught with the unknown. It is my hope that in that orientation, you can connect with a sense of resilience and empowerment to help you find your place on your path—with new awareness, intention, and commitment to your healing and wellness goals.

How to use this workbook

I encourage you to engage with the material in whatever way feels most productive and useful. In general, I have found individuals tend to get the most out of this material when they do the following:

· Read the lessons and let the information sit for a while. This information often resonates with individuals in waves, especially as they begin to notice patterns in their pain and tension in their daily lives. Allow these observations to come.

· Have a support network in place to provide in-person support (e.g., physician, counselor, licensed bodyworker). See Lesson 4 for more information about resourcing and how to use internal and external resources to support your healing journey.

· After letting the information sit, use the reflection questions as a time to write freely—without editing. The writing is just for you and often helps to bring unconscious patterns to the surface, so just let it flow and see what bubbles up.

- Try to approach your body with curiosity rather than fear. Our bodies are amazing vehicles for self-reflection—let's listen to what they are telling us.

A word on words

Sometimes words carry different meaning for people, depending on their experience and training. In recognition of that phenomenon, I want to include a few notes about some key words that we use throughout this workbook:

Pain: We use pain broadly. Pain can mean any sensation of discomfort, including muscular tension or knots, ache/throb, dull/sharp, etc. Lesson 1 will explain more about pain and how our body uses these sensations of discomfort.

Healing: We use healing to indicate the process our body experiences to be able to engage (and potentially lessen) discomfort and recover the capacity to calibrate its responses to its environment based on time, context, etc. (i.e., that was then, this is now). **Healing DOES NOT mean curing.** Our experiences, including pain, injury, and trauma, will always form a part of our memories and body experiences. Pain may be completely eliminated, and it may not be. Healing involves the ability to engage with our pain learn to manage and potentially lessen it, and restore of our ability to respond dynamically to our environment. Healing involves the ability to embrace the full scope of the human experience: pain and comfort, sadness and joy, etc. Like a single thread in the fabric of our lives, pain may be part of our story, but it is not our only story.

Visceral: When I use the word visceral, I mean both (a) physical feelings related to our "guts" or abdominal area, as well as (b) the deep, inward emotional or intuitive feelings (as opposed to the rational intellect) that some may describe as "gut feelings" or intuition.

IMPORTANT REMINDER: These materials are for informational purposes only. This book is designed to help you engage with pain that arises during the healing process after you have received any necessary medical assessment and, if necessary, treatment. The information in this book is not intended as a substitute for or a means for you to diagnose or treat medical conditions or diseases. If you have any questions about your healing process, how you're feeling (including any symptoms), or whether further assessment and/or treatment may be appropriate, please consult the proper healthcare practitioner.

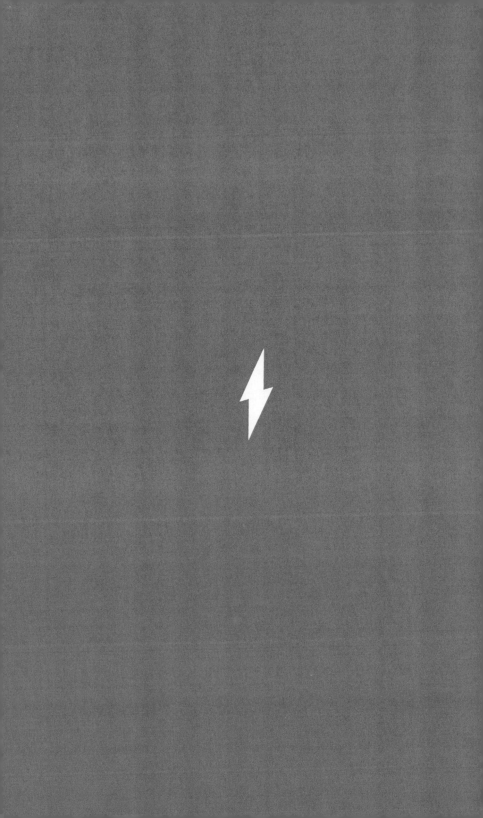

LESSON 1

CHANGING OUR RELATIONSHIP WITH PAIN

Many people seek bodywork because they are in pain. That's understandable.

Pain is, by its nature and design, uncomfortable. We also experience it in a variety of forms, all of which are designed to get our attention. It could be tension or a knot in a muscle, or feelings that are dull or sharp, hot or numb. I am grouping together all of these feelings as "pain" for the purposes of this lesson. Because pain can cause discomfort, many people come in and ask me to make that pain go away. I reply that we might not want to do that. Instead, I ask if they're willing to engage with the pain to listen to what the pain has to say. Here's why.

Pain is just information.

We have pain receptors all over our body (except in our brain tissue itself) that are activated when we perceive actual *or threatened* harm to ourselves (either physical or psychological).[1] If these receptors perceive a threat, they send out signals through our body's somatosensory nervous system to let us know that we have been or could be hurt.

The threats could be physical damage to tissue: the classic example of the pain we experience when we approach a flame.

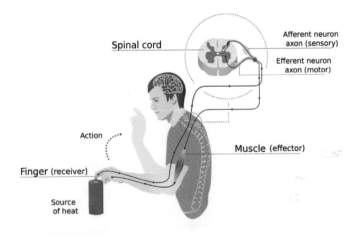

1 Van der Kolk, Bessel. *The Body Keeps the Score: Brain, Mind, and Body in the Healing of Trauma.* 2014. See also, www.wisebrain.org/ParasympatheticNS.pdf

The pain could also be caused by "psychological" or "emotional" factors. That's right—we can experience physical pain from things like "memories." In fact, neuroscience research has shown that "recalling an emotional event from the past causes us to re-experience the visceral sensations felt during the original event" and can change "brain areas that receive nerve signals from the muscles, gut, and skin."[2] To learn about how emotions can affect us physically, you can read more in Lesson 2.

The same applies to tense muscles. We have built-in alarm systems in our muscle and connective tissue (like muscle spindles) that create tension to prevent movements that may damage that soft tissue.

Either way, pain and tension protect us. Whether it's from a physical or emotional cause, the warning signals help us avoid certain movements, situations, or positions that we perceive as unsafe.

If pain and tension serve as our alarm system, why would we want to remove something that's designed to protect us?

To learn what feels unsafe, to learn why we feel we could be harmed, we have to engage with the pain and tension to learn what they have to tell us. That is how we heal. If we only look to remove pain or tension, we could be removing the very signals that are there to protect us. We may also miss valuable information and simply mask the underlying issue.

2 Van der Kolk, Bessel. *The Body Keeps the Score: Brain, Mind, and Body in the Healing of Trauma*, pg. 95. 2014.

For example, if I have a headache, rather than just reaching for aspirin and continuing about my day, I might consider another option. I might ask myself why I have a headache. Do I need to lower the coffee intake and drink some water? Have I been staring at a computer screen for three straight hours and need to move around? Is the tension in my shoulder contributing to the pain in my head?

Just to be clear, I'm not saying that pain relievers are bad or that you shouldn't look for relief from the discomfort. On the contrary, some relief from pain and tension can help us engage more fully with the underlying issue. If, however, we want to explore the possibility of healing, simply suppressing these symptoms may not be the best approach. Rather, if we can engage safely with the discomfort (rather than suppressing or masking it) to determine why we feel unsafe, pain and tension often subside naturally.

What does that mean for your bodywork sessions?

If these built-in alarm systems activate when we feel unsafe, then we need to establish relative safety in order to heal. I do that in a variety of ways in a bodywork session, and you can look for practicioners who share a similar approach.

Here are a few examples:

- I get your informed consent for a treatment plan so that you know what to expect and that you have a right to say "yes" or "no" to any techniques.

- I integrate a variety of techniques and ease into pressure and depth. That approach reinforces relative safety in the soft tissue—giving you that "body-felt" sense of safety on every level.

- It's my experience that applying those techniques slowly and gently is often more effective and efficient at helping tissue release.

- I can still go as deeply as your body will allow, AND we don't force it because I don't want your tissue to reactivate its alarm system if it feels like it may be damaged.

· When working deeply, I am OK with therapeutic discomfort but not guarding. What's the difference?

- Generally, therapeutic discomfort means you can maintain a normal breathing rhythm through the work. You may have to focus on that breathing, but you can maintain that rhythm. Guarding happens when the pain or discomfort causes you to make faces, shorten your breath, tense further, etc. If you're guarding, your body doesn't feel safe, and the work is counterproductive.

- The point is to engage with the tissue in a way that reestablishes safety—if our technique or pressure is causing more pain or guarding, then we need to back off or change the approach.

Remember, you always have the support of the practitioner to help guide you through this experience. If you're ready for it, they can help you engage with the pain or tension in a safe, productive manner. When you do that, you can help build the story and awareness of what the pain is telling us—when it hurts, when it feels better, etc.—to facilitate release and address the underlying issues.

When we engage with the pain by listening and responding to it, we can see pain for what it is: valuable information that can both protect us from further damage and help us understand its underlying cause.

FROM BROKEN TO RESILIENT

Moving from seeing pain as a sign that our body is broken to understanding it as an elegant tool our body uses to help us survive.[3]

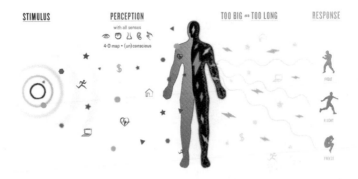

---

3 Note to reader: Remember, this mindset shift assumes that you have received any necessary medical assessment and treatment and are now working through the pain that comes during the healing process.

Questions for building your body awareness

1. Before reading this lesson, what was your first reaction when you felt pain? What did you tell yourself about your body when you experienced pain?

2. After learning more about pain in this lesson, how might you respond to your pain differently? The same?

3. What role do you believe perception and safety play in injury and healing if pain can be triggered by the perception of actual or threatened damage (physical or psychological)?

4. List some examples of when you have listened and responded to pain and tension in your body. List some examples when you've ignored or suppressed it. What circumstances contributed to the difference in your approach?

NOTES

N O T E S

NOTES

N O T E S

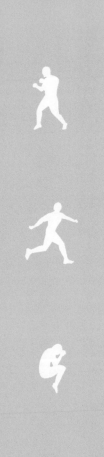

LESSON 2

HOW EMOTIONS SHOW UP IN OUR BODIES

Human beings like balance—something scientists call homeostasis. In fact, we require this balance to survive, and we don't have a big margin for error. For example, our body temperature needs to stay between 97° and 99.5° to be classified as "healthy."

Much as a thermostat keeps the temperature in a room within a close range, our bodies and minds work together to map our internal and external environment to keep us in balance—and not just for our body's temperature. This "thermostat" is called our somatosensory system.

Our somatosensory (literally "body" "sensing") system processes everything we perceive internally and externally, including sight, sound, touch, pain, etc.

If something happens that's either too big or goes on too long to push us out of balance, we respond to correct it.

You've already experienced this when you sweat. If our body gets too hot, we sweat so it cools down to the safe range.

The key is that **any** change that pushes us out of balance triggers the appropriate physiological responses to restore balance—whether that means sweating to cool us off or shivering to warm us up.

How does this balance apply to emotions?

While most people are familiar with the physical examples, the same applies to emotions and for the same reasons—to help us survive.[1] In fact, emotions "exist to be felt and listened to, for they are the signals of changing bodymind needs. They are the driving and motivating energy of the body."[2]

How?

Neuroscientists have observed that emotions actually start first with a body-felt perception of our internal environment (heart rate, breathing, etc.) and external environment

1 Damasio, Antonio. *The Feeling of What Happens: Body and Emotion in the Making of Consciousness*, pg. 54. 1999.

2 Teegaurden, Iona Maarsa. *The Joy of Feeling: Bodymind Acupressure*, pg. 55. 2003.

(touch, sound, sight, etc.). This perception is then processed through our somatosensory system and reflected physically, in the body.[3] The same somatosensory system that maps our physical environment includes the ability to track and process emotional and social cues from other people, both to protect our physical body and our relationships.

While this phenomenon has recently been mapped by Western scientists, it was also observed thousands of years ago. As one scholar of Eastern healing arts observed, "Traditional teachings say that emotions and feelings are necessary responses, natural to the human being as s/he relates to others and to the eco-system. The emotions are glandular and visceral reactions [i.e., changes in our body] to changes in the environment."[4]

Let's look at some examples of how emotions might reflect our perception of the environment and manifest in our body.

EMOTIONS AROUND PHYSICAL SAFETY

FEAR

Scientists have shown that simply seeing the facial expression of a person who looks angry can trigger a fear response in the brain and body.[5] Seeing that angry person mobilizes

3 Damasio, Antonio. *The Feeling of What Happens: Body and Emotion in the Making of Consciousness.* 1999. Note, Damasio makes clear that emotional responses appear in both the brain and the body—not just the body (see pg. 288).

4 Teegaurden, Iona Maarsa. *The Joy of Feeling: Bodymind Acupressure,* pg. 55. 2003.

5 Van der Kolk, Bessel. *The Body Keeps the Score: Brain, Mind, and Body in the Healing of Trauma,* pg. 78. 2014.

the protective "fight or flight" response in our body, causing increased heart rate, rapid breathing, etc.

COMFORT AND SAFETY

Research has also demonstrated what we have known to be true through experience of holding babies: We can also be soothed (including slowing heart and breathing rates) by something as simple as the calm tone in a voice. Before babies understand what's being said, simply using a soft, melodic tone can calm a baby.[6] The same applies to adults. In other words, when we hear that soothing voice, our body's systems perceive safety and start slowing the heart rate and breathing.

What about emotions that don't involve potential physical threats?

The same perception-response dynamic applies.

FEAR

For example, public speaking is often listed as one of the top fears people have in life. Is it because we believe the crowd will pull us from the stage and rip our limbs off? No, not physically at least. Psychologists have identified that people fear the social consequences of being judged by others.[7] We are petrified of what will happen to our job if we botch that presentation or what our friends will say if we bomb that

---

6 Porges, Stephen W. *The Polyvagal Theory: Neurophysiological Foundations of Emotions, Attachment, Communication, and Self-regulation.* 2011.

7 www.psychologytoday.com/blog/the-real-story-risk/201211/the-thing-we-fear-more-death

wedding toast. So just as when we see an angry face, our heart beats faster, we breathe more quickly, and we may start to sweat right before we get up to speak in front of a crowd.

COMFORT AND SAFETY

Similarly, scientists have found that individuals who can rely on strong, stable social support and relationships secrete fewer stress hormones and are able to better maintain health through stressful events.[8] If we know others have our backs no matter what happens, our bodies are able to remain calmer because we know the relationships that support our physical and emotional needs will remain relatively stable—regardless of the other stress we may experience.

What about feeling happy or sad for events that actually happen to other people?

Our bodies change even for events that we don't experience directly. Mirror neurons in our brain fire when we connect to the physical or emotional experience of another person or event; scientists believe these neurons form the physiological basis for empathy.[9]

Even something as mundane as watching sports on TV has been shown to cause dramatic increases in heart rate, perspiration, and testosterone levels[10]...as if the people sitting

---

8 www.wisebrain.org/ParasympatheticNS.pdf; see also Van der Kolk, Bessel. *The Body Keeps the Score: Brain, Mind, and Body in the Healing of Trauma.* 2014.

9 Van der Kolk, Bessel. *The Body Keeps the Score: Brain, Mind, and Body in the Healing of Trauma*, pgs 58-59. 2014.

10 www.nytimes.com/2000/08/11/sports/sports-psychology-it-isn-t-just-a-game-clues-to-avid-rooting. html?pagewanted=all

on the couch watching were actually playing the game themselves.

And just as our bodies respond to *any* physical change to restore balance, scientists have shown that our bodies respond to *any* change in our emotions or relationships that could throw us out of balance, whether we perceive that change to be "positive" or "negative." In fact, any major change has been shown to help predict the likelihood of someone becoming ill or suffering an injury.[11]

That means that *any* change in financial position (i.e., losing money *or* getting a raise) and *any* change in employment position (i.e., getting fired *or* getting promoted) stress our physical systems. Doesn't matter if it's good or bad, desired or feared.

How can this help you get the most out of your body-work sessions?

When you first booked an appointment, I asked you to begin to consider thinking about pain differently. Rather than approaching pain as something simply to be suppressed, approach it as useful information that can help identify the underlying cause (see also Lesson 1). That information can help you build your story around what your body needs to heal.

The emotional context forms part of your story because your emotions and your body are simply reflections of how you

11 www.dartmouth.edu/~eap/library/lifechangestresstest.pdf

perceive your environment. They form one, beautiful feedback loop that we can use to help guide your sessions.

So when you note physical responses that form part of your story, pay attention to the emotional and social context as well. As we mentioned above, emotions and feelings are responses to your perception of the environment, and those responses are reflected in your body.

For example: If your neck is really stiff, ask yourself when it gets stiff. Pay just as close attention to physical movements (when I look over my shoulder) as the social and emotional context (when my boss enters the room or when a traffic jam makes me late for work). It's all relevant because, as we've just explained, our bodies respond physically to any changes—whether those changes are physical or emotional, "positive" or "negative."

Just try to deepen your awareness of and connection with your body by noticing the how, what, when, and where of how your body feels. It doesn't have to make sense now. Just notice it and then together you can create a plan with your practitioner for how best to work with it.

In addition to noticing how you feel over time, ask yourself on the day of the appointment: How am I feeling physically, emotionally, mentally in this moment? What feels most in need of attention? How would I like to feel when I leave the session? If I want to feel "better," what would "better" feel like in my body?

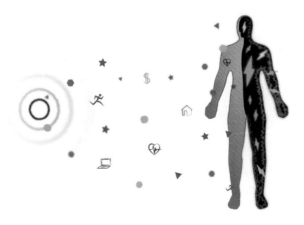

Questions for building your body awareness

1. List some examples of how your body reacts to keep its physical balance and safety. What physical sensations do you notice in your body with these reactions?

2. List some examples of how your body reacts to keep its emotional balance and safety. What physical sensations do you notice in your body with these reactions?

3. List some examples of when you have felt a physical reaction to an event that happened to someone else (i.e., if you see or hear about something).

4. If you are feeling physical discomfort, how could those reactions help you restore balance? For example, if my back tenses up when I bend over to pick something up off the floor, restricting that movement may help protect me from hurting my back more until my back feels stronger, more stable, etc.

N O T E S

NOTES

NOTES

LESSON 3

SYNCHING

LEARNING TO LISTEN, HONOR, AND RESPOND TO THE PAIN

Before we jump in, let's do a quick review. In Lesson 1, we learned that pain is simply information that helps us understand something in our body feels unsafe/threatened. Lesson 1 and 2 helped us understand that both physical and emotional events can cause physical pain.

If that's the case, then in order to heal, we need to listen and respond to what the pain has to say. By listening closely, we can gather information about why our bodies might feel unsafe/threatened and respond to those signals in a way that gives us a body-felt sense of safety and facilitates the healing process rather than hindering it.

By "body-felt," I mean what we actually feel safe on a visceral (i.e., gut) level (not just rational)—because those visceral feelings are reflected in our body. As discussed in Lessons 1 and 2, when we perceive fear, it's reflected in our bodies through signs like an increased heart rate or muscle tension. Similarly, our bodies reflect safety through signs like lower heart rate and relaxed soft tissue.

Saying or thinking we're safe helps, but it may not be what we actually feel viscerally. Those visceral feelings that are reflected in our body through heart rate, breathing, muscle tension, etc. will reveal whether our body feels safe or threatened, calm or anxious.

Most people understand this through the idea of body language. I may tell my wife I'm excited to attend her work reception (and I may really want to feel excited to support her), but if I have slumped shoulders, my eyes are on my shoes, and I stand by myself in the corner all night, my body and behavior say otherwise.

Learning how to listen to our bodies helps us identify that body-felt perception and whether there may be a disconnect between what we're thinking and what our bodies actually feel.

Why is this important?

There are two key reasons why it is critical to listen and respond to our bodies so closely:

1. The simple act of listening can actually change our body and initiate the healing process; and

2. It can help identify any underlying issues connected to the pain.

As simple as it sounds, human beings like to feel heard.

While this idea may seem simple, its importance can't be overstated. Getting back in sync with the rhythm of our bodies honors a very human, primal experience that begins when we are first born—we need this experience as babies to help us feel safe and allow our bodies to heal and grow.

Researchers have found that when a child feels heard, s/he has "a sense of joy and connection [that are] reflected in his steady heartbeat and breathing and a low level of stress hormones. His [/her] body is calm; so are his emotions."[1] They have found the same applies to adults. Simply noticing and acknowledging physical or emotional needs calms our bodies (e.g., by slowing heart rate and breathing and activating our immune system) and helps foster emotional regulation.[2]

Further, paying attention to all of the triggers for your pain (the how, when, where, etc.) helps you and the practitioner begin to identify any physical and/or emotional elements

---

[1] Van der Kolk, Bessel. The Body Keeps the Score: Brain, Mind, and Body in the Healing of Trauma, pg. 112. 2014.

[2] Ibid, pg. 273.

of the issue. Physically, if you tell me that your low back hurts when you bend to the side and twist, we will look at soft tissue that performs or supports that movement (spinal erectors, QL, obliques, etc.). Socially/emotionally, as noted in Lesson 2, if you notice that your low back also fires up when your in-laws come into town, we can work with how your body holds tension and employ techniques that may help release or cope with that tension.

How do I get in sync with my body?

1) Notice what you feel without judgment or attachment.

The nice thing is—it's simple...and in the simplicity lies the challenge!

Simply notice what you feel. Start to pay attention to the how, what, when, where, etc. of what you feel. Build out the details of your story in whatever way is most effective for you—writing, recording, drawing, etc. The key is simply to be open and approach your body with curiosity. Allow your story to unfold without worrying about making sense of it right now.

After you notice it, give yourself permission to feel it without judgment. Notice it, record it—and try not to judge it. For example, if someone got out of a chair and his back locked up, his tendency might be to say/think, "My back shouldn't hurt like that just from getting out of my chair." Maybe and maybe not. What he does know is that his back hurts when he gets up. That's it and that's enough for now. Similarly, if someone notices she clenches her jaw in traffic because she hates rush hour, she might think, "This shouldn't make me angry. This is silly." Well, it may or may not be silly, but you do know you feel your jaw clench. It's OK to leave it at that.

If you notice these judgments or any "coulds" or "shoulds" coming into your story, just put them aside and notice what "is"—a hurting back or a clenched jaw. While the "shoulds" and "coulds" can be helpful to identify possible disconnects between our thoughts and what our body feels, we just want to create some space to allow ourselves to observe and be wherever we are...even if that's having a tight back or a clenched jaw. That way, we can listen to what our bodies have to say and initiate the healing process where we actually are, not where we think we should be.

2) *Honor and try to respond to those body-felt sensations.*

At a very basic level—try to honor what your body is telling you. If you're tired, rest. If you're hungry, eat. If your jaw is clenched, try exhaling through your mouth to give it a chance to let go. You get the picture. Responding to those cues continues to deepen our body's sense that it feels heard and attended to, which deepens our connection with the body and helps facilitate healing.

I say "try to" because sometimes life happens.

Sometimes we have to wake up in the middle of the night to care for a sick child. Sometimes we have to pull an all-nighter to meet a work deadline.

If life happens, then I recommend three steps: What, Why, and How.

Acknowledge:

1) *what* you feel;

2) *why* you're not able or choosing not to respond immediately to your body's needs (I'm not going back to sleep because my kid puked in the middle of the night and I need to clean it up now); and

3) *how* and when you will address the need your body is telling you about (I'll go to bed early tomorrow and take a nap on Saturday).

From personal experience and experience with clients, taking these steps helps get through times when you're not going to respond immediately to your body's needs. That acknowledgement alone can help significantly calm the body's stress response.

MINDSET SHIFT

FROM FIX TO FACILITATE

If our body is not broken, then nothing needs to be fixed. Instead, we facilitate our own healing by learning to listen on all levels to what our bodies have to say. We can then practice giving ourselves permission to feel and connect with those body-felt experiences without judgment or attachment (and we can enlist the help of practitioners who are able to help us do the same).

How does this apply to my bodywork session?

First, you can share your story in whatever ways feel comfortable.

Helping the practitioner understand your body-felt experience and sensations can help him/her get in sync with your body and listen and respond to its needs as well.

Second, stay in sync with your body during the session.

If pressure is too deep, let the practitioner know and ask that it be lightened. If you'd like to move or stretch in a certain way, let the practitioner know and ask to move in that way.

Responding to those sensations helps our bodies continue to feel heard and safe, which can calm our bodies and allow the healing process to deepen during the session—whether that's through the activation of the parasympathetic nervous system, release of muscular tension, increased range of motion, etc. If we ignore signals like pain and continue to push through it, our body simply goes on guard and locks down to protect itself. This can stall the healing process and undermine the benefit of the bodywork. If, instead, we choose to honor the pain and ask to lighten the pressure, the body feels safe and can continue to activate its healing responses.

Eastern traditions understood the importance of this synching and facilitating process thousands of years ago and embodied the process in the term "wei-wu-wei," understood as "letting ourselves be" and honoring the "natural rhythm of things" as they are.[3] To help explain just how practitioners can help clients "let themselves be" and "honor what is," scholars recommended practitioners work with clients by "flowing like a river, reflecting like a mirror, and responding like an echo." By taking this approach, they could create a space in which clients can notice, honor, and respond more effectively to what they feel.[4]

Listening and responding in that manner will help you get the most out of the time and money you've invested in your bodywork session(s).

If you have questions about what discomfort may be "therapeutic" and what may be counterproductive, ask your practitioner. In general, you should be able to breathe comfortably during any work. If you notice yourself shortening your breath, bracing, or having trouble speaking, it's probably too deep.

And remember, listening and responding to your body can be invaluable not only because it helps facilitate healing, but because it can help you build awareness of those visceral, body-felt perceptions—whether those are of safety or fear, excitement or exhaustion. So please feel free to speak up and let your practicioner know what you need.

3 Teegaurden, Iona Maarsa. The Joy of Feeling: Bodymind Acupressure, pgs. 52, 54.

4 Ibid.

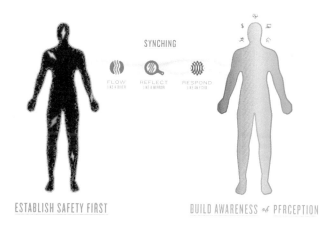

ESTABLISH SAFETY FIRST **BUILD AWARENESS** *of* **PERCEPTION**

Questions to help sync and build your body awareness

1. What do you observe about your physical discomfort? What emotions are connected to that physical discomfort?

2. Do you notice judgments pop up when you make those observations about your discomfort? If so, how do they affect your body's response to the discomfort?

3. List some examples of when you have listened and responded to your body's needs. How has your body reacted?

4. List some examples of when you have not listened and/ or responded to your body's needs. How has your body reacted?

5. If you do choose to ignore your body's needs, how can you help make sure you "balance the equation" to help address those needs in the future?

NOTES

NOTES

NOTES

N O T E S

LESSON 4

RESOURCING

BUILDING OUT YOUR TOOL KIT

Our bodies are incredibly adept at protecting us and helping us survive. If we perceive a threat (whether it's physical or emotional), our bodies protect us to help us avoid further harm. As we've discussed several times throughout the lessons so far, pain (which includes feelings like muscle tension) serves as a critical tool that our bodies use for that protection.

Why is this important? It helps us know how to heal.

Well, if you're experiencing pain, then by definition your body perceives a threat—and it wants you to stay away from what could cause you that harm—whether it's certain movements or situations. Maybe that potential harm lies in the soft tissue in the ankle that you sprained during a basketball game, or maybe it's the clenching in your chest you feel when stressed at work.

Either way, the protective response works the same—when something feels unsafe, pain and tension protect our bodies by alerting us to potential harm. Since protective responses kick in when we don't feel safe, **change only happens when our bodies do feel safe.** Our bodies can shift from defense and protection to healing and growing when we feel comfortable that further damage won't be done at the moment—whether that's putting pressure on that ankle or noticing our shoulders drop and our breathing slow at work because our boss left and we aren't afraid of being fired or berated.

So if we want to heal, we need safety. If we're going to support the healing process in bodywork sessions, we have to understand how to create relative safety for our bodies.

How can we create safety to facilitate self-empowered change and healing?

If we need to reestablish safety, then oftentimes we need some help doing it because our bodies felt overwhelmed by the threat. We have a variety of resources that can help us create safety. We use the word resources because they are general tools or assets we can draw on to function effectively, especially in adverse circumstances.

To help create safety, we can develop and draw on both internal and external resources to help establish the safety we need to allow our bodies to stabilize and heal.

INTERNAL RESOURCES

We have internal resources that can serve as incredible healing tools. We call them "internal" because they lie within our own bodies and can help change our physiology. How? The internal tools help signal to the body that it is safe so that the protective responses like pain, tension, and the fight/flight response can subside and allow the body to focus on healing the vulnerable area.

Visualization and intentional breathing are two perfect examples of internal resources.

VISUALIZATION

We are constantly creating 4-D maps of our bodies and environments. When we experience something, our brains create memories that record not only the sensations (visual, touch, taste, etc.), but also our emotional and physiological states.[1] These maps are created when we feel pain or danger, as well as when we feel relaxation and joy. When our bodies feel overwhelmed, whether that's with stress or the tension in an injured area, we can tap into these memories of joy and relaxation to help calm the protective responses and trigger the parasympathetic nervous system (the branch of our

1 Damasio, Antonio. *The Feeling of What Happens: Body and Emotion in the Making of Consciousness*, pg. 183. 1999. See also Lesson 2 in this series.

nervous system that stimulates our bodies' healing and resting responses). The more specific and detailed we can make the image, the more activated this parasympathetic system becomes—and the more we can heal.[2]

INTENTIONAL BREATHING

Intentional breathing is another internal tool we can use. Intentional breathing has been practiced across the world for thousands of years under names like pranayama yoga and hara breathing.[3] While masters practice these breathing techniques for years, anyone can begin a simple practice today with a couple of short steps.

First, close your eyes, get comfortable, and just notice your breath. As you notice the rhythm of your breathing, allow your body to breathe softly and naturally—without forcing any rhythm.

Next, as you connect with that breathing and let the natural rhythm take over, allow yourself to fully and completely exhale.

Finally, as you connect with that natural rhythm and fully exhale, allow yourself to pause slightly at the exhale before your body naturally begins to inhale again.

Breathing like this essentially signals to our bodies that it is safe to rest. While this breathing technique has been

2 To read more about the science behind visualization, read here: www.peregrinecenter.com/blog?category=Self+Care

3 See Teegaurden, Iona Maarsa. *Acupressure Way of Health: Jin Shin Do.* Chapter 4. 2003. See also Silva, Mira; Shyam Metha. *Yoga: the Iyengar Way,* pgs 154-162. 1990.

practiced for thousands of years and we know resting feels good, neuroscientists now understand that breathing in this manner helps activate our vagus nerve—the main control switch for that parasympathetic nervous system that lowers our heart rate and activates our digestive and immune systems. In other words, these breathing techniques help stimulate our resting, digestion, and healing functions.[4]

EXTERNAL RESOURCES

In addition to internal tools that help signal that we are safe, we can and need to remember that we may need external resources as well to provide support in the healing process.

While those resources could be anyone or anything, there are a few qualities an external resource must have if it is going to support the healing process. External resources need to be able to create a safe, nonjudgmental space where we have permission to feel and reconnect with our bodies without attachments, agendas, or judgments about what we should feel.

That sounds like pretty lofty stuff, but it can translate very simply.

An external resource may be a physician, massage therapist, or physical therapist who allows you to share your body-felt experience without telling you what "should hurt" or where you "should be" in your rehab protocol.

---

4 Van der Kolk, Bessel. *The Body Keeps the Score: Brain, Mind, and Body in the Healing of Trauma*, pg. 86. 2014.

An external resource could be a friend or psychotherapist who creates space for you to share your experience without having an agenda for fixing you.

An external resource can be a walking path around a lake or a pet if we can feel more connected with and grounded in what our bodies are feeling just by being in that space or with that animal.

Why is this important?

As we noted in Lesson 3, when a person feels heard (whether through active listening or synching), their brains and bodies literally change. The areas in our brain that control our fight/flight response begin to calm down, and that parasympathetic nervous system activates—initiating the systems that help us rest and heal.

By contrast, when we feel judged, we don't feel heard or supported. We feel the need to defend ourselves.

MINDSET SHIFT

FROM HELPLESS TO EMPOWERED

With increased body awareness and resources to help us safely listen and respond to our bodies, we move from feeling helpless to empowered. No longer feeling quite so whipped around by pain and discomfort, our increased body awareness and sense of safety enables us to make informed choices about what action will align with our healing goals.

What does this mean for your bodywork session?

Your practicioner can draw on this information in your sessions to help activate your body's healing responses. You may build and hone your internal resources and connection with your body through exercises like visualization and intentional breathing.

I also recommend you search for practitioners who embody the qualities of an external resource by creating a safe space for you simply to notice and feel whatever it is you feel—without an agenda. Further, I also recommend confirming what other external resources you have to support your healing process. After all, you will likely be spending between one and two hours with a practitioner that week, and you have a lot of time out in the world living your life. Look for practitioners who can help you brainstorm about what other resources you can use to find support.

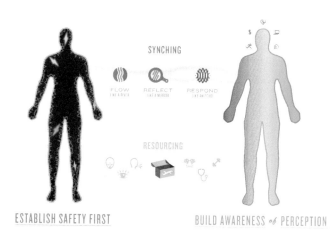

ESTABLISH SAFETY FIRST   BUILD AWARENESS of PERCEPTION

Questions for building your resources and body awareness

1. Take 10-15 minutes and practice this visualization exercise. Try to think of a time or experience when you felt relaxed, calm, and comfortable. Try to get as specific and detailed as possible with that memory. For example, if you remember sitting on the beach, close your eyes and remember how warm the air felt on your skin. Was there a breeze? What did the sand feel like beneath your toes? Did you have a drink in your hand? What sounds do you remember (ocean waves, music, birds, etc.)? Really try to reconnect with every sensory experience that forms part of that memory. After you have a detailed sense of the memory, notice what you feel in your body when you work with this visualization exercise. How do your muscles feel in your legs, shoulders, and face? What do you notice about your heart rate and breathing rhythm?

2. Take 10–15 minutes and practice the breathing exercise. What do you notice in your body when you focus on breathing?

3. In addition to breathing and visualization, are there other internal resources that you draw on? If so, list them and describe how your body feels when you connect with these internal resources.

4. List 3–4 external resources you have that meet the criteria of being safe, nonjudgmental resources that help you connect with your body-felt experience. What do you notice in your body when you're with these external resources?

5. What additional resources, if any, would you like to put in place to support your healing?

NOTES

N O T E S

NOTES

N O T E S

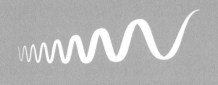

LESSON 5

OSCILLATION

OR WHY HEALING AND RUNNING A MARATHON ARE SIMILAR

Let's do a quick review of the steps we've learned so far so that we can better understand how oscillation fits in.

1. *Your body is not broken—pain and tension are survival responses.*

   As we saw in Lesson 1, pain and tension are natural, adaptive responses designed to protect us from something that our body perceives as unsafe (whether that threat comes from a physical or emotional source).

2. *We need to reestablish safety by synching and resourcing.*

    Since our body reacts to protect itself from perceived threats, healing requires that we create relative safety. We do that by listening and responding to the signals from our body (Lesson 3—Synching) and drawing on the internal and external support we have (Lesson 4—Resourcing).

Once we've synced with our body and established our resources, how can we engage with the vulnerability to help our body relearn how it can be safe and strong?

That's where oscillation comes in.

We need to build capacity steadily over time through a process of engaging areas that may feel unsafe and then resting and recovering to allow our bodies to integrate the gains.

Why do we need to do this over time?

Healing is not linear. We may feel good one day and sore the next—even after a bodywork session or PT. Why?

It's just the way our bodies function.

Healing essentially involves building capacity in our soft tissue and nervous system. We are relearning how to be strong where we once felt unsafe. Building that capacity takes time and requires breaks to rest and recover.

For me, the best analogy to the healing process is training to run a marathon. For those unfamiliar with marathon training, search the Internet for "free marathon training program," and you will see for yourself.

If you want to build the capacity to run 26.2 miles, the training is not linear.

You do not run 1 mile on Day 1, 2 miles on Day 2, 3 miles on Day 3, until you run 26 miles on the 26th Day. Instead, here's how the training would go:

- you have long days (10- or 15-mile run, but never over 20 miles)

- you have short days (3 miles)

- you have easy days (light jogs)

- you have hard days (faster paced)

- you start shorter and slower and build to longer distances (runs may be 3 miles to start, 20 miles at the end), and don't forget

- you have **REST days**—days specifically set aside to allow your body to rest

This combination helps your body acclimate over time so that your soft tissue and nervous system learn how to process the stress that comes with running 26.2 miles.

The same applies to the healing process.

You are helping your body and mind build the capacity to feel safe and strong where it once felt unsafe (whether that's rebuilding strength in a sprained ankle or being able to stay grounded when talking to your boss without experiencing that stress response).

The process not only happens over time, but it can also happen within a single training or bodywork session. For example, here's what oscillation may look like during the synching and resourcing process of a bodywork session. If a client is describing his pain and feels ready to engage more deeply with it, I may spend time helping him develop a very detailed, body-felt sense of the pain (e.g., Is the pain hot/ cold? Dull/sharp? Where does it start and stop in the body?). Once the client has this detailed body-felt experience of pain, oftentimes I will shift and have him focus on a place of comfort. The client will then go through the same process of developing a detailed body-felt experience of comfort (e.g., Does the comfort feel warm/cool? Full/empty? Where does the place of comfort start/stop in the body?). After building that detailed sense of comfort, we may go back to the pain to see how/whether it has changed, or we may stay with the comfort if the client feels like he wants to rest.

Alternating between the feelings of pain and comfort can help a client realize both consciously and unconsciously (i.e., rationally and on a body-felt level) that experiences other than pain, including rest and comfort, may be both possible and accessible.

The process of alternating between work and rest, pain and comfort, challenge and recovery is called oscillation, and it can be a crucial step in the healing process.

So how does this apply to the healing process?

Sometimes it is hard to tell when to push it and when to rest.

That's why even with free marathon training guides out there, athletes hire coaches. Coaches serve as important external resources to help tailor the program to meet the athlete where s/he is every day. That means even if the program calls for a long run, the coach might suggest skipping the run and resting if the athlete feels too sore.

For your healing, you can call on practitioners to help coach/ guide you through the process.

Remember, you're recovering from something that your body felt was overwhelming enough to use pain or tension to protect itself. As a result, it's completely normal that you may need to lean on external resources from time to time for support through the process.

MINDSET SHIFT

FROM AVOIDANCE TO ENGAGEMENT

Rather than looking to avoid or suppress pain, we can engage safely with it—learning where our body perceives a lack of safety. We can allow our bodies to heal at their own pace, using synching and resourcing to listen and respond to our needs while reinforcing relative safety. As part of that process, we can honor when we feel ready to work and when we need to rest—understanding that we build capacity over time in a nonlinear manner.

How does this apply to your bodywork session?

Look for trends over time.

Since this process is not linear, it becomes even more impor-tant to look for trends over the course of four to five appointments and keep in mind what else is going on in your life.

You may feel better one day than another or better after your first session than your third. Sometimes we have stress or lack of sleep due to other causes in our lives, and sometimes our body just needs a little extra time to rest.

The point is the same: We are not made of switches that can be flipped to make us heal—any more than we can flip a switch and run 26.2 miles.

Our bodies have incredibly complex, interconnected systems that work together to keep us alive. When we heal, we need to reestablish the balance and function of all of those systems—that's why they call it a healing process.

Looking for trends over time allows our bodies time to integrate the work and experience the normal ups and downs of life. It also helps us make a better determination whether the work (bodywork, PT, etc.) is helping or whether we need to refine the treatment plan.

This nonlinear nature of the healing process can test our patience and resolve more than any tender trigger point or grueling workout.

Why?

Because it acknowledges the truth that the exact trajectory and timing of healing is unknown. It acknowledges that there are no magic formulas. No silver bullets.

The best we can do is use our understanding of how our bodies and minds function so that we can create a space that facilitates healing...honoring that each individual's process is unique and moves at its own pace. We simply need to listen and respond to our bodies so that we can allow that process to unfold.

The good news is that when we create that space and honor the process, we often heal more quickly than if we try to force it.

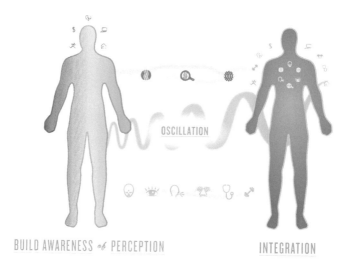

BUILD AWARENESS *of* PERCEPTION   INTEGRATION

Questions for understanding oscillation and building your body awareness

1. Reflect and get a detailed body-felt sense of a time when you were joyous. What does your body feel like? Now, reflect on a time and get a detailed body-felt sense of a time when you were sad. What does your body feel like? Now, go back and reconnect as fully as possible with that feeling of being joyous.

2. Over time, have you felt progress in your healing process? If so, when? Over time, have you experienced plateaus or setbacks in your healing process? If so, when?

3. How easy or difficult has it been to let your body heal at its own pace? Why?

4. What internal/external resources can help you determine when to push or rest in the healing process? How do they do that?

N O T E S

NOTES

N O T E S

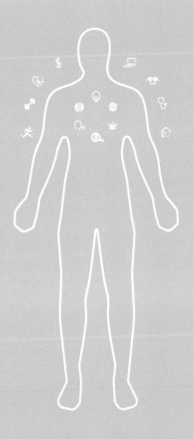

LESSON 6

INTEGRATION

...AND WHERE YOU GO FROM HERE

Congratulations—you've come a long way.

You've invested the time and resources to help you get to know yourself and your body.

You've deepened your understanding of your body's protective mechanisms and the role pain and tension play in helping you survive a potential threat to yourself—whether that's physical or emotional. (Lessons 1 and 2)

You're synching—building awareness of how your body feels without judgment. You're giving yourself permission to feel and building the story of when and what makes it feel better or worse. (Lesson 3)

You're resourcing—developing the internal and external tools to support you in the healing process and help your body feel safe again. (Lesson 4)

You're oscillating—engaging with the vulnerability safely, alternating between work and rest, challenge and recovery. This oscillation is helping your nervous system and soft tissue build capacity over time—relearning how to be strong in areas that once felt vulnerable. (Lesson 5)

It takes incredible courage to engage with pain and tension so that you can learn the tools to help yourself heal. Simply moving from avoidance to engagement with that pain and building awareness helps people move from feeling helpless to feeling empowered since they understand the pain and its role and can make decisions about what next steps will best serve their goals.

These shifts from broken to resilient, avoidance to engagement, fix to facilitate, and helpless to empowered help people experience significant growth physically, emotionally, and spiritually during the healing process. For that reason, I see the healing process as a journey—a journey that I believe embodies the idea of a pilgrimage in the classic sense of that word.

Parker Palmer defines a pilgrimage as:

> ...a transformative journey to a sacred center full of hardships, darkness, and peril. In the tradition of pilgrimage,

those hardships are seen not as accidental, but as integral to the journey itself. Treacherous terrain, bad weather, taking a fall, getting lost—challenges of that sort, largely beyond our control, can strip the ego of the illusion that it is in charge and make space for true self to emerge. If that happens, the pilgrim has a better chance to find the sacred center he or she seeks. Disabused of our illusions by much travel and travail, we awaken one day to find that the sacred center is here and now—in every moment of the journey, everywhere in the world around us, and deep within our own hearts.[1]

I can't think of a better description for what the healing process is like and how we grow because of, not in spite of, the challenges that the process presents.

So what now? How can I use this information?

There are a couple of steps you can take to help you integrate this growth experience and use it going forward.

1.   Appreciate it—embody it.

As you saw in Lesson 4, our emotional and physiological states form integral parts of our memories just like sights and sounds do. These emotional and physiological memories can serve as future internal resources—tools that you can use to remind your body that it has felt and can feel healthy and strong even when pain or tension arises.

Synching means listening and honoring the full scope of our experience: pain and relief, sadness and joy, etc. So take some time to get a good body-felt sense of the "healing" or

1 Palmer, Parker. *Let Your Life Speak: Listening for the Voice of Vocation*, pg. 18. 2000.

"growth" you've experienced. Create a detailed memory of what healing or growth feels like in your body. Breathe into and connect with these feelings. What do you notice in your body? Is it warm/cold? Open/full? Build a detailed story of what healing and growth feel like in your body and get as specific as possible.

Doing this also helps us take stock of how far we've come, which is important. Oftentimes we move directly on to the next area of pain or struggle—immediately shifting our focus to the next thing we want to change. Taking the time to appreciate and embody these feelings acknowledges the hard work we've put in, how much we have grown, and just how resilient and supportive our bodies can be. Enjoy it.

2.   Keep some perspective…these feelings don't last forever.

Simply put: Life happens. I don't have a crystal ball, but I feel pretty safe in betting that at some point you are going to experience something else that will test your limits—physically, emotionally, or spiritually.

It's actually a good thing.

As psychologist Mihaly Csikszentmihalyi notes in his book *Flow*, humans are naturally drawn to increase our capacity and evolve.[2] His research aligns with ancient Taoist philosophy, which recognized that "each aspect of the self tends to seek growth, then a new balance or stability, then more growth, and so on. The urge to growth is the urge to

---

2 Csikszentmihalyi, Mihaly. *Flow: The Psychology of Optimal Experience.* 2008.

wholeness."[3] Growing is just part of being human, and sometimes we experience growing pains.

So if we're naturally drawn to experiences that test our limits, developing awareness and tools to meet these ever-increasing challenges can help keep us grounded during the process—even when it's uncomfortable.

So the next time something stressful comes up and challenges your physical, emotional, or spiritual capacity, the hope is that you remember a couple of things:

1. You're not broken.

    When you experience pain or tension, remember that it is helpful information. It's a sign that your body is incredibly adaptive and protecting you.

2. Get in sync with it.

    Give yourself permission to feel. Listen, honor, and respond to those body-felt experiences without judgment. Our body's feelings (physical and emotional), whether they are pain or relief, joy or sadness, provide useful information about our body-mind needs. Listening and responding to those feelings helps initiate the healing process and create awareness around what you need.

3 Teegaurden, Iona Maarsa. *The Joy of Feeling: Bodymind Acupressure*, pg. 49. 2003.

3. Resource.

It's completely normal and appropriate to need and look for resources and support to help you through the process—in fact it's encouraged. Something that causes pain or tension is your body's way of saying "I don't feel safe." By definition, it needs some support to reestablish that safety and to heal. Remember, you have both internal and external resources to help guide you through this experience. Use them.

4. Oscillate.

It takes time for your body to build the capacity to feel strong where it felt unsafe. Listen to your body and allow for the process to evolve at your body's own pace—not someone else's. Work when you feel strong. Rest when you feel tired. The oscillation is how our body heals, restores balance, and builds capacity in all of its systems.

5. Healing is a pilgrimage.

Healing is not linear and can often contain hardship and challenges. The experience of engaging with those hardships and challenges like pain, tension, or uncertainty serves as the catalyst for growth and building new physical, emotional, and spiritual capacity. Remember, you already have those qualities and the potential for that capacity inside you. It's simply about creating the space to allow them to emerge.

PAIN

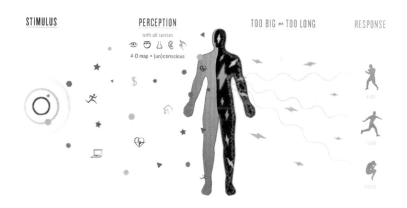

STIMULUS   PERCEPTION   TOO BIG *or* TOO LONG   RESPONSE

with all senses

4-D map • (un)conscious

HEALING

SAFELY ENGAGE VULNERABILITY

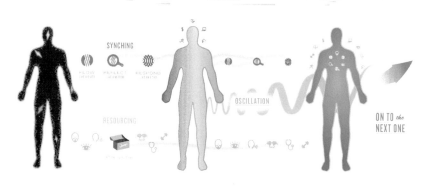

SYNCHING

OSCILLATION

RESOURCING   ON TO *the* NEXT ONE

ESTABLISH SAFETY FIRST   BUILD AWARENESS *of* PERCEPTION   INTEGRATION

BROKEN *to* RESILIENT   FIX *to* FACILITATE   HELPLESS *to* EMPOWERED   AVOIDANCE *to* ENGAGEMENT

MINDSET SHIFT PROGRESSION

FROM BROKEN TO RESILIENT

FROM FIX TO FACILITATE

FROM HELPLESS TO EMPOWERED

FROM AVOIDANCE TO ENGAGEMENT

Questions for building your body awareness

1. What have you learned about yourself as you've moved through these lessons?

2. What changes have you noticed in your body as you've moved through your first bodywork sessions and read these lessons?

3. Are there areas that need more time/space for you to listen and honor that they may not be ready for change?

4. What questions do you have about this process, bodywork, or the material?

5. What are your next steps?

N O T E S

NOTES

N O T E S

RESOURCES

The science underlying the mind-body connection

If you're interested in the underlying science behind the mind-body connection, I have listed some initial texts below, many of which I cited in this workbook:

Damasio, Antonio. *The Feeling of What Happens: Body and Emotion in the Making of Consciousness.* 1999.

Levine, Peter, PhD. *In an Unspoken Voice: how the body releases trauma and restores goodness.* 2014.

Porges, Stephen W. *The Polyvagal Theory: Neurophysiological Foundations of Emotions, Attachment, Communication, and Self-regulation.* 2011.

SomEx: Experiential Healing Center. This group of psychotherapists in Memphis is doing some fantastic work incorporating somatic (body-based therapy) into their counseling work with trauma and addiction. You can learn more about them at ehcmemphis.com.

Teegaurden, Iona Marsaa. *Acupressure Way of Health: Jin Shin Do.* 2003.

Van der Kolk, Bessel, M.D. *The Body Keeps the Score: Brain, Mind, and Body in the Healing of Trauma.* 2014.

I also write periodically on the mind-body connection on my blog, located at peregrinecenter.com/blog.

ACKNOWLEDGEMENTS

First, thank you to my wife, Heather, and my children for supporting me as I've gone through my own journey of injury, pain, and healing. It hasn't always been easy, or pretty, or quick, and you've stuck by me and supported the work I've done, including the work on this book. Thank you for keeping me grounded and loving me.

Next, I want to thank Mindy Oldham. For helping me gain a more embodied sense of the concepts in this book, and the power of this work, and the potential beauty in the healing process. For the countless lunches and meetings discussing the theory, the practice, and the course we teach together on Holistic Bodywork for Injury and Trauma. Your teaching, support, and feedback, including editing help, have been invaluable to the creation of this book, the course, and my own development. It is also just incredibly fun to work and brainstorm with you.

Thank you to Mary Beth Crawford whose immense amount of guidance and wisdom have encouraged and facilitated my pursuit of this work, which has become a calling.

Thank you to Sharon Prete whose coaching and wise counsel have supported me on my own pilgrimage. Your support on my journey and willingness to discuss this work have helped me refine my understanding of the concepts in this book and develop both personally and professionally. Thank you.

Thank you to Cumberland Institute and all the teachers there for the incredibly thoughtful training. I've been to a lot of schools, and that was the best training I've received—hands down. Special thanks to Steve Sommers for his teaching at Cumberland and in the Jin Shin Do training, which has been invaluable to my personal and professional development and become a foundational element of my work.

Thank you to Tim Delger for all of his excellent work on the graphics and layout for this book. His work took complex theoretical concepts and translated them into useful images—and the incredible graphics speak to his talent. Thank you to the McKinney sisters (Aretha, Margaret, and Nicole)—you all have supported me and my curiosity in this work in so many ways over the last decade that this work feels like a natural evolution from our conversations.

Finally, thank you to my clients, for their willingness to allow me to listen and support their efforts to do this work—I learn from you every day. Choosing to engage in this type of work is not easy, and your courage inspires me every day to continue my practice and my own journey.

ABOUT THE AUTHOR

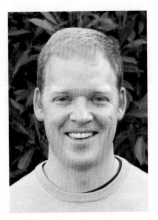

Michael Stahl is a licensed massage therapist (LMT), an educator who teaches health practitioners how to work effectively with injury and trauma, and the owner of the Peregrine Center, a holistic bodywork center in Nashville that provides therapeutic, integrative bodywork to clients of all ages and physical abilities. He has trained in multiple soft tissue techniques, including neuromuscular therapy (Trigger Point), acupressure, myofascial work like Active Release Therapy, and Swedish massage. His current teaching schedule includes professional education classes and client workshops such as: "Holistic Bodywork for Injury and Trauma" and "Anatomy, Physiology, and Kinesiology for Level 1 and 2 Iyengar Yoga Teacher Training."

He's also a lawyer, having earned his law degree from Stanford University and his undergraduate degree at Georgetown University. Prior to pursuing law, he also earned a master's degree at Vanderbilt University as a graduate fellow.

While not the usual career path, the decisions and direction of Michael's career have been guided by a natural curiosity, passion for learning and growth, and a simple question, "What's possible?" Michael's passion to discover what is possible regarding pain and healing began when, at the age of 15, he fractured his spine, which resulted in serious nerve damage and led to subsequent injuries. Michael immersed himself in anatomy, physiology, physical therapy, and anything else that might help him recover. Through this experience, he began to ask himself and others "What's possible" with respect to pain and the healing process. You can learn more at peregrinecenter.com/staff.

When you ask yourself what's possible, your natural curiosity about yourself and your challenges becomes clear, and that's when growth, healing, and realization of your full potential can begin.

That question—asking more of himself while helping his clients see their potential—has shaped Michael Stahl's career path and the clients he's helped serve.

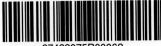

Made in the USA
Lexington, KY
30 December 2018